CHIROPRACTIC LIVING

A PAIN-FREE, STRESS-FREE, INJURY-FREE LIFESTYLE

TABLE OF CONTENTS

One of the most sought after forms of alternative healing is chiropractic care. Amongst cancer survivors who seek chiropractic therapy, 84% do so to alleviate pain, improve mood and sleeping habits, as well as to relieve stress.

The human body is designed to move and movement requires varying amounts of stability and motion. When movement occurs, patterns of stability and motion can occur in efficient or inefficient ways. As structures accommodate movement, the load placed on everything from joints to muscles and tendons to nerves changes and these changes can produce symptoms. In the process of wanting to avoid symptoms, the body will often develop compensation patterns. A common result of this compensation process is the feeling of being 'tight' or 'tension'. This tension serves a protective role, thus it is referred to as protective tension.

The development of protective tension and the reason behind its presentation is one of the least understood mechanisms in musculoskeletal care. The body is smart enough to constantly monitor loads and prevent excessive load of any given structure to ultimately help prevent injury. If you are feeling 'tight', there is a reason and your body is sending you a signal. However, many people will ignore this signal until more pressing issues develop, such as pain. So how does one handle a muscle that 'feels tight'? Unfortunately, the solution is not as simple as just stretching. Stretching often provides temporary relief because of underlying joint dysfunction, stability and/or mobility deficits, or muscular weaknesses that need addressed.

Thinking Beyond Stretching

To illustrate this concept, let's look at the classic example of someone with 'tight hamstrings'. The common solution many people hear from coaches, trainers, medical professionals, and the all-knowing local gym guru is, "You should stretch your hamstrings more." So the well-intentioned individual chooses to stretch their hamstrings more often because they feel they have received good advice from someone they perceive as knowledgeable.

However, the majority of people will eventually find themselves in a cycle of temporary relief from stretching. They stretch, feel better, then some time later they feel tight again. So they stretch more and more, but fail to have any sustainable results all because they received very poor advice from the start. Be critical of your information source. Just because someone owns a Mac doesn't mean they are qualified to be a programmer for Apple. Get the point?

The purpose of chiropractic treatment is not only to relieve pain, but to improve quality of life by alleviating systemic problems relating to muscles and the central nervous system. Given the researched benefits of chiropractic care, it is likely that you or someone you know could benefit from this alternative therapy.

Let's take a look at the top reasons you might benefit from chiropractic care.

1. Elevates Sports Performance

Both athletes and non-athletes can benefit from sports-specific chiropractors. These specialized doctors have a focus on manipulating joints, soft tissue, and the spine to improve recovery time and prevent injury of strains, sprains, and even concussions.

As a Chiropractor i can teach you how to focus on the proper techniues for the sport you play. This will include stretching techniques which can reduce the occurrence of an injury, the severity of an injury, and a recommended rehabilitation time frame for healing.

2. Reduces Headaches

Do you have freuent headaches? Do you find that headaches dramatically impact your health and ability to maintain the lifestyle you want? Neck pressure and movement can exacerbate the severity

f headaches caused by abnormal head positioning such as hunching over at a computer during the work day.

Chiropractic therapy can remove obstructing structures causing the tightness in the back and strain on the spine. Receiving chiropractic care is an effective way to limit the occurrence of headaches, and lessen the intensity when they do occur.

3. Stimulates the Immune System

The immune system interacts directly with the nervous system affecting overall health. Again, obstructions with the signaling pathways between the nervous and the immune system impact the ability to heal adeuately.

Without the use of surgery or medication, chiropractic care removes these barriers so that the body can properly repair itself at a genetic level and stimulate the immune system fully.

4. Wellness and Prevention

Chiropractic procedures manipulate the spine and entail a variety of procedures which treat underlying health problems. For instance, decompression exercises improve sleeping habits and have no known side effects.

5. Alleviates Allergies and Asthma

Both chiropractors and parents of children suffering from allergies such as asthma support the positive results of chiropractic treatment.

Studies also support that chiropractic therapy benefits patients by decreasing the amount of medication needed. They suffer fewer asthma attacks and report an overall lessening of symptoms leading to an improved quality of life.

6. Pregnancy

Throughout pregnancy, many women experience chronic back pain due to the changing weight distribution on the pelvis and joints. Pain and muscle spasms may increase the likelihood that a pregnant mother will struggle during labor and delivery.

Chiropractic treatment focuses on balancing the muscles, pelvis, and ligaments during pregnancy to relieve pressure on the uterus. This treatment increases the likelihood that the child will be born via a preferable position while lowering the risk of being born through cesarean section.

Seventy-two percent of women report finding relief from pain during pregnancy and labor resulting from chiropractic care. Part of this success may due to the fact that women are encouraged and shown how to follow a proper exercise routine for pregnancy. This reduces weight gain, improves hormones, and allows for a more comfortable rest during sleep.list-of-chiropractic-therapy-benefits

7. Mitigates Chronic Pain

Low back pain affects more than 10% of the population globally, and is the most common occupational injury in the United States and Canada. North America ranks low back pain sixth amongst contributing factors for increased medical cost. Compared to conventional health management practices, chiropractic care is low cost and improves the healing of the entire body.

Doctors of chiropractic also focus on education, which is critical to reducing injuries, disability, care costs, and adverse side effects. Chiropractic therapy is also a patient preference for providing pain relief.

8. Manages Behavioral and Learning Disabilities

Chiropractic procedures improve wellness and can help reduce hyperactivity and disruptive behaviors linked to ADHD and learning disabilities associated with autism.

Evidence supports that chiropractic treatment can better able a child to concentrate. In turn, it improves learning and behavior by limiting causes of agitation.

9. Weakens Dependence on Medication and Medical Interventions

There has been a 65% increase in patients seeking spinal treatment over an 8 year period, contributing to a significant rise in healthcare costs. However, approximately 96% of people with low back pain can find relief without surgery. This could lead to a remarkable lowering of costs.

Chronic pain is on the rise. The first line of treatment most individuals turn to for pain relief involves medication. Tens of thousands of people consuming drugs like acetaminophen and oxycodone have reported injuries and deaths directly resulting from drug use. Drugs have adverse side effects unlike chiropractic care.

Young adults are especially susceptible to drug overdoses. Dr. Joseph Wiley, Chief of Pediatrics at Sinai Hospital in Baltimore, is quoted as saying "If you extrapolate from an adult dose to a pediatric dose, you may be right…you may be wrong."

10. Normalizes Blood Pressure

Hypertension affects around 33% of Americans. Most of these individuals will use medication to manage the condition. Chiropractic care can significantly control blood pressure. Chiropractic adjustments have been shown to result in a decrease in both systolic and diastolic blood pressure readings.

In fact, tests show that chiropractic care works as effectively at managing hypertension as do two of the most commonly prescribed medications. Chiropractors focus on the bone at the top of the neck in proximity to the brain stem which may be the reason for the impact on regulating blood pressure

Discovering the reason behind your tight muscle is a complex process.

Here are just few common reasons why tight muscle develop protective tension:

1 – Poor Posture due to Weakness of the Abdominal and Glute Musculature

anterior_pelvic_tiltThe anterior pelvic tilt is a common posture seen today. As the pelvis rotates forward due to stability and muscular control issues, this places stress on the hamstrings since they attach directly to the pelvis. Not only is this a static posture consideration, but also applies to dynamic posture or essentially the posture one assumes while moving. Movement will place greater stress on the anterior and posterior abdominal slings. These slings serve as a link between your shoulders, spine, and hips. Weakness in their ability to control pelvic and spinal movements, such as rotation and extension, can create overactive or tight hamstrings. In this case, the hamstrings will continue to feel tight until the underlying issue of correcting posture and pelvic/spinal stability are improved.

2 – Adverse Dynamic Tension of the Sciatic Nerve

grays-sciatic-nerve-anatomy-image-IIPeripheral nerves, such as the sciatic, have their own uni⬚ue biomechanics to allow for movement of the arms or legs. Nerves are surrounded and encased by muscle/connective tissue, so they need to be able to 'slide' through tissue during movement. If they can't slide, tension develops because nerve tissue is highly sensitive and can be injured very easily if too much stress is applied to it. Hamstring tightness can be attributed to the sciatic nerve or its branches, the tibial and common peroneal nerves, being entrapped within the hamstrings and/or calves. The detection of neural tension requires specialized training. Those that are qualified utilize specific soft tissue work and neural mobilizations tailored to treat neural tension.

3 – Accumulation of Adhesive Tissue within the Hamstrings

imagesThis is common in athletes and runners because of repetitive use. Adhesive tissue can develop within musculature in response to overuse, thus affecting how a muscle contracts and lengthens. Typically a muscle that does not lengthen appropriately will create the feeling of tightness. Again, specific soft tissue work is tailored to treat adhesive tissue and allow for proper hamstring function.

4 – Joint Dysfunction of the Pelvis or SI Joints.

Abnormal joint mechanics will alter muscle function. If joint centration or how the joint moves is altered, this will alter length-tension relationships of muscles surrounding the joint. This affects muscle function and will potentially place tension on the hamstrings. These are best addressed by joint mobilizations or adjustments/manipulations. Licensed chiropractic professionals are well trained in identifying abnormal joint mechanics and the impact it has on the body and nervous system.

How do weaknesses develop in the first place? Stress, trauma and overuse shut down the connection between the brain and muscle rendering muscle contraction less efficient and effective. This connection is necessary for proper muscle function. Net effect is your muscle won't contract when you need it to or may not contract at all. This may not seem like a big deal but wait until one weakness stacks on to another and the entire functioning of your body is affected.

Most people are shocked to find out that not all their muscles are contracting perfectly. The objections I hear are: "But I work out!" Or "I feel fine!" How can we function if this is the case? The reason we get around so well is that our nervous system finds ways to work around the weaknesses. Like a road closure that makes you take the long way around, the 'detour' your body takes to avoid the weakness isn't as efficient, may look odd and could even be causing imbalances at your joints that render activity painful. Over time joints can easily get worn out when muscles aren't doing their job to support and protect them. At the end of the day, even though we are compensating, it gets the job done and that's all we really care about until we are so injured and uncomfortable that we can't do something. Then we look for solutions.

One very effective solution for muscle imbalance is Muscle Activation Techniꝗues. In a treatment, the MAT specialist will find out what you can't do and test and treat all the muscles that perform that function. Once the muscles are activated, a MAT specialist will retest and make sure all the muscles that help you perform that function are strong and stable. They even get you to stress your body out during a treatment to see if the muscles they treated stay strong. This gives them information they need to help you get stronger, faster.

Once a Muscle Activation Techni?ues Specialist gets muscle function back, your joints are more balanced taking the stress off of them and for many, decreasing pain and stiffness. Post treatment mostly everyone reports feeling different when they walk. They also observe feeling looser, more agile and the complaint they came in with typically changes in ?uality and severity. The way your body feels improves gradually over the course of treatments and you begin to feel relief. Many clients do not return because the problem they came in with is gone.

Muscle activation techni?ues can be used for natural pain relief treatment. They can also change unhealthy movement patterns and restore muscles and joints to a healthier condition.

Muscles may feel painful and sore for many reasons:

*They may be overworked.

*They may be stressed due to poor posture and misalignment.

*They may be fatigued or strained from repetitive movements.

When muscles become overworked or strained, imbalances arise. Some muscles are getting stronger, but others weaken.

Modern muscle activation rooted in ancient pain relief therapies.

Several modern styles of muscle activation are practiced around the world, but some of their characteristics are not new.

Applied Kinesiology (AK), and a spin-off version of AK called Touch for Health, were mainly developed by chiropractors. During an AK session, the practitioner will determine if some muscle groups have weakened, causing others to compensate. They will apply touch and resistance to muscles, to stimulate underworked muscles and energy systems.

Modern reflexology is founded in similar principles. Points in the feet, hands, and ears are said to correspond to other muscles, organs and physical systems. These channels through which energy flows to vital organs, muscles and other parts are known as meridians in far Eastern medicine. A practitioner presses on reflexology points to stimulate the flow of energy and improve health along meridians.

Both AK and reflexology are examples of modern therapies with ancient roots. Far Eastern medicine has included these concepts and practices for centuries.

Acupressure and acupuncture, for example, are rooted in activation. After assessing the medical condition of their patient, the practitioner determines which parts of the body need more healing energy and which areas need less. They use pressure or pins to conduct energy toward weak or understimulated areas, and to draw energy away from overworked areas.

What is muscle activation for pain relief and healing?

The techni2ues described above share a common element. They redirect energy in the body, for healing purposes.

When muscles feel painful or tense from workloads, then often one set of muscles is overworked while another should be working harder.

By applying muscle activation methods, we shift energy away from overworked muscles and send it to weak or underworked muscles.

Once the practitioner has used their activation techni2ues, they assess how the muscles responded. If the underworked muscles became more active, then the muscles should work in better balance. Pain should be relieved, new patterns of activity can develop, and the client can practice habits to prevent pain long-term.

In a nutshell when you get a MAT session the specialist will find out what you can't do, restore proper muscle function and reinforce those habits and motions that will speed healing. There is no therapy like MAT so if you've tried many other things with limited success or if you've just been injured and are wondering if MAT is right for you, contact a MAT specialist and find out. They treat the muscular system and many physical challenges can be alleviated simply by getting the largest organ of your body working properly.

Gluteal activation

Gluteals are the group of muscles comprising of your buttocks. Out the four muscles in your buttocks, there are only 3 groups of muscle that can be found on your buttocks. These muscles are gluteus maximus, medius and minimus. The fourth group which is the smallest one is the tenor fasciae latae muscles that can be found in the anterior area of the body. Functioning together, the gluteal muscles handle most of the motions of the upper leg, which includes rotation of the thigh, and abduction and turning of the hip.

Among the 3 gluteal muscles, the gluteus maximus is the biggest as well as the nearest to your skin. Beginning near the top of the hips and affixing over the upper area of the femur, it is this thick, broad muscle that provides the glutes its contour. The gluteus maximus works numerous essential features in the leg and pelvic regions. For example, it helps in the expansion of the leg and the turning of the hip joint in addition to allowing the body to elevate from a sitting down position by tugging back the hips.

Subsequently in descending sequence of dimension is the gluteus medius. Much like the gluteus maximus, which partly covers it, this muscle group is thicker and starts at the higher pelvis. It takes up considerably less surface area than the bigger muscle, but, and terminates at the higher trochanter, a backward-extending outcropping of the femur identified just beneath the head of the bone tissue. The gluteus medius is vital to thigh assistance during strolling and hip flexion - when people walk, this muscle tissue facilitates the weight of the body as it is positioned on the thigh, therefore maintaining the pelvis from tipping away from the weight-bearing calf. Furthermore, every time the hip is flexed or prolonged it helps in twisting the thigh.

Most minuscule among the list of gluteal muscles is the gluteus minimus. This particular muscle is situated underneath the gluteus medius. It comes at the outer fringe of the mid-pelvic area and wraps up, like the gluteus medius, at the greater trochanter. The majority functions of the gluteus minimus are carried out in assistance with the gluteus medius; it helps, for example, in thigh spinning and the flexion of the hip.

Stress to the gluteal muscles caused by overly vigorous physical activity can lead to soreness in Tension to the gluteal muscles as a result of excessively brisk physical exercise can result in tenderness in the area. There are a variety of stretches that will help calm gluteal discomfort and tightness. Lying on the back and tugging your legs up to the chest one at a time, for instance, can alleviate soreness in the gluteus maximus. The gluteus medius and gluteus minimus could be expanded by lying down on the back, bending your knee, and traversing the curved leg on the opposite leg, utilizing the hand to carefully drive the knee towards the ground

It's hard to overemphasize the importance of gluteal training for back pain prevention and overall well-being. The gluteal muscles - particularly, the gluteus maximum and medius muscles - are needed for back and pelvic stability.

Unfortunately, hours of sitting each day has left many of us with weak, overstretched gluts. This causes a number of different problems in the body. These muscles help to stabilize the sacroiliac (SI) joints, which form where the hip bones meet the sacrum; their weakness can cause hypermobility in the SI joint, leading to lower back pain and potentially sciatica. The gluteus medius helps to stabilize the pelvis, particularly when our weight is on one leg. The gluteus maximum has connections with the thoracolumbar fascia, a connective tissue that attaches to several other muscles throughout the core, and with muscles in the lower back that help to hold the upper body upright. When the gluteus maximus engages, so do these other muscles and tissues, creating spinal stability. When the muscles of the buttocks don't engage, others may be slower to engage, thereby creating spinal instability.

Yet another way in which glut weakness affects the lower back is by calling on muscles in the back to compensate for its jobs. Normally, the muscles in the buttocks engage when we extend the hip or rotate the leg outward; if they can't achieve this task, then muscles in the lower back, along with the hamstrings in the back of the thigh, will have to take over. This can cause strain, spasms and muscle knots in the overworked muscles.

When muscles go unused for a long time, the brain stops sending signals to fire them because it has learned to redirect the signal to other, compensatory muscles (this is an instance of muscle memory). Rewiring this memory requires that you do simple, targeted glut activation exercises first, then, once the muscles have "remembered" how to fire (really, once the brain has relearned to fire them), you move on to integration exercises, which teach your body to fire the gluts along with other muscles they're supposed to work with.

Activation and Integration Exercises

Activating the gluts can be done with simple exercises like bridges, the side-lying hip abduction exercise (also called "the clam") and the quadruped hip extension. More complex integration exercises that work the muscles in the buttocks as well as others throughout the core are lunges, bridge variations, plank variations and deadlifts for the gym-goers.

Changing Habits

The best way to maximize your maximus and medius is to sit less in conjunction with exercising more. It will be much harder for your brain to learn to fire your buttocks muscles if they're being compressed for most of the day. If you work at a desk, be creative and find a way to raise your work surface so you can stand for part of the day.

Lower back pain often stems from another source, such as the buttocks. A strong rear end is a crucial component of back pain treatment and prevention

Inhibition of the gluteal muscles

Low back pain has been associated with inhibition of the gluteus maximus. The activation of the gluteus maximus during hip extension is delayed in people with a history of low back pain compared to people with no back pain. In people with low back pain hip extension is initiated by the hamstrings and erector spinae instead of the gluteus maximus. Even after the episode of low back pain has resolved, the altered firing patterns in the gluteus maximus remain.

Janda described a similar pattern of delayed activation of the gluteus medius during hip abduction in patients with low back pain .

People suffering from ankle sprain injuries also have been shown to have reduced activation levels of the gluteus maximus .

The gluteus maximus plays an important role in maintaining an upright standing position. Lengthened gluteal muscles as a result of our sitting lifestyle leads to a decreased stabilizing function in the gluteus maximus.

Inhibition and delayed activation of the gluteus maximus compromises pelvic stability. This can result in compensation by the lower back and more altered muscular firing patterns and function. In the case of low back pain, ankle and probably all lower body injuries, rehabilitation needs to focus on re-activating the gluteal muscles.

Weak or inhibited gluteal muscles contribute to injury

Weak or delayed activation of the gluteus maximus and gluteus medius is a root cause for many injuries and chronic pain.

Hamstring strains: Due to delayed gluteus maximus activity, the hamstring muscles become dominant during hip extension, which can cause hamstring strains [10]. A lot of athletes that pulled a hamstring keep suffering re-injuries despite their focus and efforts to strengthen the hamstrings. They are reinforcing a compensation pattern instead of reactivating their inhibited glutes. Shirley Sahrmann said, "Any time you see an injured muscle, look for a weak synergist." A synergist is a muscle that performs the same joint motion.

Low back pain: Gluteus maximus activation plays an important role in stabilising the pelvis during the task of lifting. Delayed gluteus maximus activation also causes excessive compensation of the back extensors.

Anterior knee pain: The excessive internal rotation of the femur as a result of glute weakness increases the pressure on the patellar cartilage.

Anterior hip pain: Decreased force production from the gluteus maximus during hip extension is associated with increased anterior translation of the femur in the acetabulum. The increased femoral anterior glide could lead to increased force and wear and tear on the anterior hip joint structures

Lower-body malalignment: Weak glutes results in increased internal rotation of the femur, knee valgus and foot pronation

Gluteal weakness also has been associated with anterior cruciate ligament (ACL) sprains, chronic ankle instability, and iliotibial friction syndrome

Serratus anterior activation

The serratus anterior muscle is found on the sides and back of the torso on both sides. It is made up of several smaller muscles, giving it a serrated, or toothed appearance, and its primary function is to stabilize and affix the scapula, or shoulder blade, to the chest wall. If its function is impeded, the scapula may lift off the chest wall during certain maneuvers with an appearance of wings -- known medically as "winged scapula.

The serratus anterior muscle is actually a collection of separate muscles that arise from the anterior, or front, side of ribs one through eight or nine, depending on the individual. This attachment occurs just past what is known as the mid-axillary line, or the line running down from the center of your armpit, medically known as your axilla. At the other end, the serratus anterior muscle inserts into the anterior aspect of the medial border of the scapula -- or the front facing side of the middle edge of the shoulder blade.

Structure

The muscle is called serratus anterior due to its attachment, and due to its structure. As it is made up of eight segments in a typical person, it has a serrated appearance much like that of a serrated knife. It is possible to observe this looking in the mirror with your arms raised. The lateral thoracic arteries supply blood to the serratus anterior muscle, and the long thoracic nerve arising from cervical vertebrae C-5 through C-6 in the neck provides its nervous system connection.

Action

The purpose of the serratus anterior muscle, like that of any muscle, can be derived directly from its attachments: Its action is to hold the scapula, or shoulder blade, against the back and to stabilize it while you use your shoulder. Specifically, it abducts and upwardly rotates the scapula -- pulling the medial aspect of the scapula forward and up. This serves to anchor the scapula against the chest wall during abduction of the arm, when the arm is pressed back as in a pushup.

Dysfunction

If either the nervous supply or blood supply to the serratus anterior muscle is sufficiently interrupted, through either trauma or tumor invasion, this can cause a condition known as winged scapula. In order to test for this condition, a medical professional watches a patient perform a standing pushup maneuver against a wall. If there is dysfunction of the serratus anterior muscle, the medial edge of the scapula will lift off the back of the chest wall on the affected side, giving the appearance of a wing

A winged scapula can be serious, but it depends on the causes. There can be two main types of "injuries" that could cause you to have a winged scapula. Both of the injuries have to do with your serratus anterior. A muscle which its job is to "glue" your shoulder blade towards the midline so it doesn't "wing-out" during shoulder movement:

What are the causes?

It could be NEUROLOGICAL, a nerve issue.

The most serious and rare reason is an injury to the nerve that activates the serratus anterior muscle. If you are suffering from nerve damage (which again, is rare) your muscle will lose its ability to contract. Therefore, there will be a winging on the shoulder blade as the muscle is unable to keep it "glued" to your back.

There are 17 different muscles that attach to your shoulder blade. At times it is not just an injury to the long thoracic nerve but an injury to other nerves that come from your neck that will lead to it. A big sign is if your winged scapula is very noticeable on overhead movement.

The most common cause is weakness

Weakness in the muscles that stabilize the shoulder blade will cause your scapula to move where it should not move. It will give you the appearance of a winged scapula.

Common therapy procedures are targeted towards strengthening the serratus anterior. However, sometimes the exercises that are prescribed are not efficient at solving the issue because the problem is usually more complicated than just a weakness of one muscle.

Furthermore, if the body does not know how to activate the right muscle it will compensate and use the wrong muscles to get the task done. So you might think that you are working out your serratus anterior but other muscles are taking over and the exercise is ineffective.

A common complaint is heard:

My right scapula pops out of my back continually, despite how much I work my serratus anterior; which I'm told is the cure. How can I fix my problem?

The treatment needs to be targeted towards proper muscle activation and postural correction. If your chest muscles are too tight from rounded shoulders, the shoulder blade will constantly be pulled out of alignment. If there is a rotator cuff injury, it needs to be addressed as well.

Tight shoulders are highly correlated to this condition, find out if your shoulders are tight

Fixing a winged scapula tends to be more complicated because it greatly differs from patient to patient. It could be a nerve, the shoulder blade muscles or like many times a combination of the two. You need a full movement analysis to determine the pattern that causes or aggravates the condition. Moreover, the exercises that are actually going to help fix the issue.

You need a full movement analysis to determine the pattern that causes or aggravates the condition and more importantly the exercises that are actually going to help fix the issue.

have yet to meet a chiropractor who is not looking for a universally applicable step-by-step treatment approach to help patients reclaim and transform numb, tingling, tight, stiff or painful body parts so they can feel, in each moment, wholeness and well-being.

However, after 28 years in practice, I don't think there is such a step-by-step treatment approach. I think we develop individual treatment approaches or processes depending on the chiropractor, the patient and the circumstances.

My current treatment approach includes using manipulation/mobilization, warm laser, deep muscle stimulator, fascial release, foam rolling, stretching, muscle activation, core work, and whole-body exercises (often utilizing bands and kettlebells).

Now let's connect what we see in the winged scapula to the corrective exercise strategies we can prescribe for this dysfunction. Please keep in mind that the best exercise you select for your client is the exercise that produces carryover, meaning it improves movement capacity and movement quality, in this case of the scapula.

Postural Analysis of Scapular Winging

Static postural analysis may reveal scapular winging. However, I use many tests to determine what the scapula is doing functionally. Let's consider some possible scenarios:

- Winging may be noted during glenohumeral joint flexion.

- Winging may be noted during glenohumeral joint abduction/elevation.

- Winging may be noted during the return from glenohumeral joint elevation, most notably during the first half of the movement from 180 degrees to extension.

- Winging of the entire medial scapula border may be noted on the push-up "plus" movement pattern test challenge.

If you see scapular winging in the static posture evaluation, have the patient elevate the arm maintained in external rotation. Elimination of scapula winging confirms posterior instability.

The scapula is also probably winging if you get stuck in the bottom position on the bench press, in which case you need serratus anterior strengthening work. (This can be accomplished with military press work and incline front raises.)

Scapular winging during any of these movement assessments indicates a mechanical defect of an underactive serratus anterior (SA), a long serratus anterior nerve dysfunction or a motor coordination problem. The SA is considered a global stability muscle of the scapula. The serratus originates on the profound side of the medial border of the scapula and passes to attachments on the first nine ribs. The serratus pulls the scapula inferiorly and laterally; the rhomboids pull the scapula superiorly and medially. A chronically shortened or overactive serratus will pull the scapula wide on the posterior rib cage, causing the rhomboids to be strained long. This pattern frequently accompanies a kyphotic thoracic spine.

A winged scapula is often associated with overactive pectoralis minor muscle length. A short pectoralis minor muscle (a common postural finding) pulls the scapula forward and down by tilting the scapula anteriorly. The corocoid process moves anteriorly and inferiorly and the inferior angle of the scapula moves posteriorly. It produces medial rotation of the scapula (downward rotation of the glenoid). This explains how the overactive pectoralis minor muscle alters the scapular movement. Palpation of the pectoralis minor muscle will demonstrate tenderness if it is overactive. The shortening of the pectoralis minor is related to SA and trapezius muscle imbalance. This imbalance is one scenario responsible for patients with impingement syndrome. Part of the scapular winging treatment plan is correcting the muscle length-tension of pectoralis minor.

Exercises to Improve Scapular Winging

If there were a set program for all scapular winging patients, we would have found it by now and scapular winging would be rare. I suggest you use some of these exercises as a base, observe the response over a couple of weeks and act accordingly. Teaching awareness of proper scapular position is first. Train normal scapular alignment in the seated, standing, wall lean and Ruadruped positions.

Push-Up / Serratus Plus: The "push-up plus" or "serratus plus" seems to be the most popular exercise used to strengthen the SA muscle. To properly perform this exercise, the patient needs to know these tweeks: 1) In the push-up position, place the thumbs together. 2) Lift the hands slightly above shoulder height (the hands should be under the eyes) and add slight internal rotation. 3) Just move the shoulder blades, don't move the head or drop the hips. 4) Push the scapula apart, let gravity push them back together again, push the scapula apart (that is one repetition). If the patient can't get into a push-up position, start them out on the forearms.

In my experience, doing "push-up plus" variations is the Ruickest way to correct a weakness. For example, progress to reaches from prone-on-elbows; reaches from a plank position cause more weight to shift into the SA and cause reflex stabilization. Moving from prone-on-elbows to the start position of a push-up also has deep developmental roots from a sensory standpoint. I like to have patients perform a downward dog (yoga position) and add a push-up plus between each downward dog. This helps produce stabilization through better perception in the core and shoulder girdle.

Band or Cable Chops and Lifts. The chop is performed by attaching tubing or a cable at a high point of attachment and holding both handles. Kneel at an outward angle with the outside knee down. Both knees should be flexed at 90 degrees. The patient should narrow their base to within 6-inch width of knee of one leg and heel of the other. Hold hips directly under the trunk and spine erect with the shoulders back and scapula properly placed. Arms should be extended with palms facing together while holding the handles. Pull the tubing down and across the chest while keeping it close to the body. Shoulders should turn minimally and the head should face forward. All actions should be done with the arms. The tubing should come across the body from shoulder to opposite hip, palms facing down. Tubing should be in line with the closest arm. Before starting the exercise, make sure the scapula are set properly.

The lift is performed with the tubing at a low point of attachment. The patient should grab both handles and kneel at an outward angle with inside knee down. Both knees should be flexed at 90 degrees.

Incline Push-Ups: Use a power rack to perform incline push-ups on a barbell. Patient should start with the body at the lowest incline that doesn't allow their shoulders to wing, which means placing the bar relatively high. Perform three sets of between eight and 12 repetitions. As they become stronger and learn to control their scapular motion, they can work their way down the rack until they're doing regular push-ups with perfect body alignment.

Serratus Punches: I have prescribed serratus punches in the supine position, the standing position, with hand weights, without hand weights, with tubing and with cable. This is one exercise you just have to tinker with until it achieves the desired effect of activating the SA.

Shoulder Scaption: Every chiropractor should know shoulder scaption because it has such overall benefits for all kinds of shoulder conditions. Holding a light pair of dumbbells (1-5 lbs), the patient stands with the arms in the scapular plane with the thumbs down. As the arms are raised, they begin to rotate externally (thumbs begin to rotate outward). By the time the arms are at shoulder level, the thumbs should be facing up. The elbows stay straight throughout the exercise.

Competitive swimmers train an average of ten to twenty thousand yards per day. At eight to ten arm cycles per twenty-five yards, this leads to nearly one million shoulder rotations per week. It's no wonder studies have shown the lifetime incidence of shoulder injury in competitive swimmers is over 70%.

The most common shoulder injury incurred in swimmers is "swimmer's shoulder." This syndrome is a combination of any of the following: rotator cuff or bicipital tendonitis, subacromial bursitis, shoulder impingement, and glenohumeral joint instability. It is not simply a condition of overuse; the repetitive use must be combined with some other aggravating factor, such as supraspinatus or biceps avascular tendinosis, impingement syndrome, labral injury, or instability due to ligamentous laxity or muscular dysfunction.

Muscle Imbalances and Scapular DysfunctionThe most common problem leading to swimmer's shoulder is a weak serratus anterior. This increases the rhomboid activity, which leads to anterior impingement of the biceps and supraspinatus tendons. The serratus anterior also attaches to the scapula, which is the link in the kinetic chain from the legs and trunk to the shoulder. In fact, scapular dysfunction is present in 68% of all rotator cuff problems. For every two degrees the glenohumeral joint moves, the scapula should move one degree.

ImpingementImpingement occurs when the soft tissues of the subacromial space (supraspinatus tendon, tendon of the long head of the biceps, and the subacromial bursa) are compressed between the head of the humerus, the coracoacromial arch, and the anterior acromion. Inflammation of these tissues worsens the impingement. Impingement is common in swimmers, volleyball players, baseball pitchers, and tennis players, due to increased overhead movements. Poor flexibility in the shoulders can lead to increased impingement symptoms.

It is also caused by prolonged postural stresses, such as sitting at a computer for work.

Shoulder LaxityThe rotator cuff holds the humeral head, preventing anterior and superior movement. Common causes of instability are shoulder hypermobility, increased internal rotation and adduction strengths, overuse, overuse of hand paddles while swimming, technique flaws, and decreased core strength. Instability leads to subluxation, and, combined with repetition, leads to inflammation and pain, which leads to scarring, which leads to more inflammation, pain, and dysfunction.

Prevention and Rehabilitation: Technique ChangesSwimming technique needs to incorporate body rotation with core strength, early catch, early exit, and straight-through arm pulls. Thumb-first hand entry stresses the biceps attachment to the labrum, leading to impingement. Hand entry that crosses the midline leads to anterior impingement. Asymmetric body roll and unilateral breathing both cause a compensatory crossover, which increase the risks of impingement. Proper, symmetrical body roll decreases most impingement risks. Other technique contributors are improper head position, forward shoulders, and scapular instability (see Strengthening section). Stretching, proper warm-up, and preventive strengthening must also be incorporated into practices.

Prevention and Rehabilitation: StrengtheningStrengthening, both for injury prevention and rehabilitation, must focus on stretching the strong groups of muscles and strengthening the weak ones. Shoulder injury is prevented first by core stabilization and then by scapular stabilization. Strengthening should focus on endurance of the serratus anterior, lower trapezius, and subscapularis, as well as taking into account the strength ratio of the internal and external rotators. Stretching should focus on the pectoralis major and minor, the posterior shoulder capsule, and the latissimus dorsi. Core strengthening should focus on the lower abdominals and increased pelvic control.

Exercises to include in a swimmer's routine include: scapular elevation with the thumbs up and arms thirty degrees forward; push-up plus; rowing with scapular retraction and palms rotated up; reverse push-ups; unilateral shoulder shrugs; horizontal abduction; and shoulder abduction. Sport-specific exercises include ball throws with a rebounder, punching, and PNF 2 maneuvers. Athletes can also use an ergometer to work these muscles. These exercises should be done with low weights, 1-3 sets with 25-30 repetitions, or to fatigue. When these exercises can be done without pain, gradually increase the weight in one-pound increments. This routine should be done either after swimming, or as an isolated workout session, to decrease injury risk. Core strengthening exercises can be done any time.

For the internal and external shoulder rotators, isolated exercises have been shown to emphasize better muscular recruitment. If the external: internal rotation strength ratio is

70-80%, focus on internal rotation strengthening. If it is less than 70%, focus on the external rotators. When the ratio is 60-65%, replace the isolated movement with dynamic exercises, such as pull-ups, latissimus dorsi pull downs, overhead presses, reverse pull-ups, and push-ups. All of these exercises will enhance glenohumeral stability. They should be done with 3-7 sets of 8-15 repetitions, with 2-4 minutes of rest between sets.

ConclusionApproaches to prevention and active rehabilitation of swimmer's shoulder are essentially the same: correct improper technique; stretch the tight musculature of the chest and anterior shoulder; strengthen the core musculature and the scapular stabilizers; and reduce strength imbalances in the shoulder rotators. Coaches and rehabilitation providers need to work together with these athletes in order to prevent future injury and correct problems that may already be present.

Thoracic mobility

Injuries to the thoracic spine – the twelve vertebrae and surrounding tissue that make up the mid-back – are less common than injuries to the cervical or lumbar spine. This is due to the relative stability of the thoracic spine, which is fairly rigid and attached to the ribs and breastbone. Still, thoracic spine pain is not unheard of, and when it happens, can be unpleasant.

Some conditions that can cause pain in the thoracic spine include ruptured discs, scoliosis, degenerative disc disease, protruding discs, and arthritis of the spine. The most common causes of injury to the thoracic spine are strain from lifting heavy objects, or accidental injury from a traumatic event, such as a car accident or sports injury. When thoracic spine pain is present, some people may choose to try chiropractic care as an alternative treatment to, or in conjunction with, traditional medical care.

How Chiropractors Treat Thoracic Spine Problems

No matter what your condition, a chiropractic treatment plan will begin with an initial consultation with the chiropractor. During this initial meeting, the chiropractor will take a complete medical history, a thorough description of the symptoms the patient is presenting with, and make an examination. Tests such as x-rays and MRIs may also be ordered to help facilitate or confirm diagnosis. Once a diagnosis has been decided on, the chiropractor decides on a treatment plan, which is then executed over a series of sessions.

Specific techniques used in chiropractic treatments of thoracic spine ailments include:

Adjusting from the prone position, where the patient lies flat on his or her stomach on an adjusting table.

Adjusting from a supine position, with the patient lying flat on his or her back.

Incline adjusting, where the chiropractor uses a bench table with attachments that allow it to be raised to a 45- or 50-degree angle.

It is important to remember that, although these techni ues may bring some relief to thoracic spine conditions, chiropractic cannot fix a herniated disc, foraminal stenosis, or other spinal injuries. Also, you should consult with a physician before beginning chiropractic, or any other form of alternative therapy.

If conservative treatments do not alleviate your back pain, contactchiropractic concepts pte ltd (Singapore) to learn how our minimally invasive outpatient procedures can help you rediscover your life without back pain.

Chiropractic Care for the Thoracic Spine

The goal of the chiropractor treating a patient for thoracic back pain will usually focus on reducing the pain and inflammation in the area. The treatments may include:

- Spinal adjustments

- Specialized exercise recommendations

- Ergonomic training

- Distraction

- Heat or ice

- Traction

- Electrical stimulation

The chiropractor may also recommend nutritional supplements like proteolytic enzymes to aid in managing the swelling and pain that may be caused by disc herniation and some other back injuries. They may also recommend dietary changes or weight loss to help the patient manage their pain.

Chiropractic is a safe, effective, non-invasive treatment for mid to upper back pain. Many patients experience results immediately which is another draw for people. Most patients with back problems will be advised to maintain regular chiropractic visits in order to effective manage the pain and keep it at bay.

Posture

Dedicating some time to improving posture is a very smart way to help reduce your overall injury risk as well as help give yourself a much more confident, lean appearance. Individuals who are making an effort on a regular basis are going to find that over time it's something they have to think about less and less as it eventually grows to be an automatic reaction they have when they feel as though they are slouched over.

We have all heard it before, "Sit up straight! Don't slouch!" If you're like most people good posture can slip out of your daily habits. From time to time we may remember to sit tall while at the desk or to not slouch while waiting in line, but the reality is that we forget about good posture. It seems like by the time we remember our lower backs are already aching or we have neck pain. I will discuss how small adjustments during your day will lead to improved posture alignment. We will discuss the importance of good alignment and exercises you can do to improve your posture imbalances.

Posture consciousness is a fun way to give thought to your body alignment. When I work with my clients I always start by explaining body alignment and I start with the core. The core of the body has three pillars. Pillar one is the shoulders, pillar two is the mid-section wrapping all the way around from front to back, and the third pillar is the hips. Aligning your three pillars will ensure proper posture and prevent injury during exercise. When I instruct my clients to engage their core they know to engage the three pillars by;

(1) pulling their shoulders back in line with their hips

(2) pulling the core in tight-even below the belly button

(3) lining up their hips with the shoulders. Hearing the verbal queue of "3 pillars" is a quick and easy way to assess posture and get in check.

It is critical to have good posture because it allows necessary air flow to circulate throughout the body. This alone enhances energy levels by providing oxygen for cellular respiration. Proper posture also decreases the risk of injury and improves self-confidence. How is your posture? Do you think about it during the work day? What about while you workout? If you rarely give thought to this topic then I suggest making small reminders. Yellow sticky notes on an outlook agenda is a great way to set reminders. You want your eye to catch the reminder and then engage the three pillars quickly. Before long you will make it a daily habit. When making posture adjustments try talking yourself through the verbal core activation above using Pillars, 1, 2, and 3: Shoulders, Abs, and Hips. Say it in your head as you activate and you will immediately improve posture. You will appear slimmer and have a stronger core which decreases your risk of back pain. It is a great trade-off for posture consciousness.

If you are experiencing current pain in the lower back, neck and shoulder areas due to posture I always recommend an evaluation from your practitioner. If you are interested in preventing or correcting back/neck pain or are interested in improving the strength and conditioning of your core, then check out the exercises below. You can perform these exercises as pre-hab, which is done at the beginning of the exercise session.

Remember when your grandmother told you to sit and stand with good posture or else you'd get stuck in a slouched position? Grandma was correct with her focus on good posture. As a chiropractor, I treat many people who have less than ideal alignment and structure. The majority of their postural issues can be directly attributed to lack of focus on correct posture. What I routinely see is people with forward head posture and forward rolled shoulders. This is an easy condition to acquire because most people sit at computers, work at a desk or slouch for the majority of their work and school days.

Having key muscle imbalances will cause a person with poor posture to not be able to "fix" their own malformations because their spine and joints get stuck in positions which are not natural. When a person has weak, underactive muscles coupled with tight and overactive muscles you have a recipe for structural disaster. When one has postural imbalances with inappropriate muscle firing patterns a person will not be able to "sit up straight" no matter how hard they try. For example, a person suffering from forward head posture and loss of cervical spine lordosis will feel tension in their posterior neck muscles if they try and hold their neck in the correct postural position. This is not a sustainable thing to do as it's not comfortable and the muscles will eventually fatigue in the neck region.

This is where Chiropractic and Physical Training are essential. The objective of a savvy personal trainer and chiropractor is to help our patients' correct postural imbalances through realigning the spinal joints and by retraining the muscles, tendons and ligaments to support the spine in the correct ways.

The importance of having good posture is often underestimated. When one has chronically bad posture for a sustained period of time, the muscles become fibrotic and weak. This leads to a spine which degenerates much quicker than it was designed to. These are things nobody needs to experience in life. Below are some key exercises that will help retrain ones posture.

External Rotation: Choose light weight and keep the elbows tucked in in an L shape. Rotate forearms laterally until you hit resistance. Keep elbow tight against the body throughout the movement.

How to Improve Posture

This used to be something we all practiced in elementary school but over the years, the practice has pretty much died out. There are several simple exercises that you can do to improve your overall stance, and take some of the pressure off of your lower back and spine. The first one, done while sitting on the floor, is a simple one. Sit with your back against the wall, with your legs straight out in front of you. Slowly roll a medium-sized ball from your lap to your feet, without moving either leg, or bouncing yourself to reach the end. Move as slowly as possible. The purpose of this is to slowly decompress your spine, strengthen your back muscles and improve your flexibility. Do this for about five minutes or 10 repetitions.

Stand Up Every Hour

The first thing that will be very helpful towards improving posture is making an effort to stand up at least once every hour. When we spend long periods of time sitting, we're more likely to get more and more comfortable in our chairs, essentially shrinking down as time goes on.

By standing up, you help lengthen the body once again, so when you go back to the sitting position your posture is that much better. If you have to, set a timer to go off on your desk to remind you to get up and move around. The movement will also help energize you so you can think clearer when you get back.

Practice Deep Breathing Exercises

Secondly, you also want to periodically check your breathing as well. When we are taking very shallow breathes we're going to reduce the expansion of our rib cage and lungs, which significantly changes our posture.

By deep breathing at least ten times every few hours or whenever you think about it, you'll help oxygenate your blood, providing more energy and helping you feel refreshed. By nature, when we take a deep breath our posture automatically improves, so this is a very simple way to improve posture quickly.

Stand Against A Wall At Least Once A Day

A simple yet very effective technique for improving posture is to stand against a wall and notice how much of your back is touching it. Ideally, almost the whole spine would be pressed up against the wall, and there would not be any major space, particularly around the lower back region.

If you can place a whole fist behind your lower back, this is a strong signal you're really using a sway back position and need to work on lifting up the hips more while squeezing the stomach.

Consider Getting Regular Massages

Finally, the last step you can take for improving posture is to really think hard about getting regular massages. These will really help to reduce your overall stress level, which is vital to ensuring you maintain proper posture.

When we're heavily stressed out, we are going to tense up our shoulders, causing neck and shoulder pain.

Another simple exercise to improve your posture is a classic one. Find a large book that can easily be balanced on your head. Stand with your back flat against the wall, and reach up with both hands to place the book on top of your head. With your arms down by your sides, slowly pace across the room, keeping the book as evenly balanced as possible. You will notice, as you do this, that if you slouch your shoulders forward or let your chin dip down, the book will slide off. Practice these things every day, and you will see improvement in both your stance, and your pain

By keeping all of these points in mind and including them regularly throughout your day, improving posture will be something that's easily accomplished by you in a short period of time

Want to learn more about how your posture can affect your health? The dedicated professionals at the Chiropractic concepts pte ltd (Singapore) care about you and want you to be in the best shape possible

Nutrition and diet

Many people do not consider the role of nutrition in their physical health, but when you stop to consider it, nutrition is an integral part of health. If you are receiving chiropractic care, your chiropractor may work with you to ensure that you are eating a proper diet that contains fresh fruits and vegetables, whole grains, lean meats, low fat dairy and healthy fats.

If you have a poor diet compounded with bad eating habits, your body will not operate to its optimal efficiency which will make you feel tired all of the time. As a result of this inefficient operation, your body will start to break down. If you tend to eat a lot of processed foods, sugar and empty calories that have no real nutritional value, you are setting yourself up for inflammation. Inflammation leads to severe joint pain among other painful health conditions.

When a person is being treated by a chiropractor, they can maximize the effect of the treatments that they receive by adopting a good self-care routine. The routine should include regular chiropractic treatments, optimal nutrition, proper hydration, a reasonable amount of exercise and plenty of rest.

If you are unsure about what kind of foods you should be eating, speak to your chiropractor who can probably give you some good information on what to eat. When in doubt, consider consuming raw foods dense in nutrients, especially vegetables.

Among the many things that a chiropractor recommends to a patient, a healthy diet is most important. A proper diet is essential to heal the proper-diet-hanson-chiropractic-everett-wa-minspinal cord, along with prevention of further damage.

According to a study conducted in the state of New York, chiropractors were asked if they used any nutritional counseling in their treatments, which not just includes back problems, but also obesity, artery diseases, diabetes and a variety of other diseases affecting the human body.

Around 80 percent of those surveyed stated that they did use some form of nutritional counseling in their treatments, which gives an overview of the importance of proper diet in chiropractic. 50 percent of those who used nutritional counseling considered it to be a very important part of the chiropractic therapy.

The Link between Chiropractics and Diet

Chiropractic therapy treats numerous ailments, such as inflammation in the lower back or autoimmune anomalies like arthritis, scoliosis, neuritis or osteoarthritis. Research suggests that dietary changes can affect inflammation, which in turn can reduce the symptoms and pain caused by it. Also, as most chiropractic patients are women, other symptoms that they may suffer from, such as menopause and premenstrual syndromes, can also be cured by proper diet and nutrition.

Not only that, but a proper diet can also help prevent spinal diseases from developing. As obesity is one of the most common causes of back problems, eating healthy non-fat foods can make a person less prone to spinal diseases like Sciatica.

There are numerous benefits in keeping a healthy diet, including increased energy, lower blood pressure and improved cognition, which result in a speedy recovery. Health foods such as low sugar whole grains, fruits and vegetables also reduce the risk of spinal tumors and cancer

Here are some of the benefits of various foods:

Fresh vegetables including cabbage, peppers, carrots, spinach, kale, tomatoes and legumes are foods that are high in fiber and contain minerals and vitamins required by the body. You should aim to eat 7 – 9 servings of fresh vegetables daily.

Fresh fruits in season including strawberries, red grapes, blueberries, cherries, blackberries and pomegranates are loaded with high levels of antioxidants which help the body to get rid of toxins and free radicals.

Whole grains such as whole wheat bread, oats and brown rice are good choices that help the body to function with fiber and valuable amino acids.

Fresh herbs (when possible) and spices can not only add flavor to food, but provide a good benefit to the person consuming them. Turmeric contains a large concentration of anti-inflammatory compound that is easily digested. Cinnamon, cider vinegar, basil, mint, chamomile, parsley, chili pepper and black pepper all contain compounds that reduce inflammation.

If you are not eating well, your nerves can be affected by impacting their ability to share information. Improper nutrition can affect the body's ability to repair muscle, muscle density, the function of your organs and fluid levels in your cells.

When you eat well, your body runs at its optimum best, making it an efficient machine. When you eat well and nourish your body in conjunction with chiropractic care, you increase your chances of successful treatment. Whole food nutrition increases your body's health including the health of your nerves, connective tissues and muscles. As you improve your nutrition, you may find that you need fewer chiropractic adjustments.

Reduce Inflammation With Diet

Another factor of poor diet is altered pH levels, such as increased acidity within the body. This can stimulate the nerves that sense pain, increasing discomfort. The pH levels are made more acidic by eating grains, meat and cheese.

Fruit and vegetables, in particular white potatoes and spinach, promote a more stable, less inflammatory state.

Long-term acidity can potentially lead to weakened bone and chronic pain syndromes.

There is also mounting evidence that free radical activity and inflammation play a fundamental role in the development of many conditions and diseases, including painful joints and muscles, rheumatoid arthritis, osteoporosis, Type II diabetes, obesity, cardiovascular disease, respiratory diseases, periodontal disease, reproductive complications, auto-immune disorders, some forms of cancer and dementia.

All these conditions have been linked to levels of free radicals in your body – if levels are high, this indicates that the body is under oxidative stress, which adversely affects the body's immune defences and leads to high levels of inflammation and damage to cells and our DNA.

Free radicals are produced within the body every time we breathe in oxygen or pollutants, are exposed to sunlight or exercise.

Antioxidants fight free radical activity, protecting your cells and your DNA and reducing oxidative stress.

To protect cells against free radical damage you should increase the level of antioxidants in your body.

You can boost your antioxidant level, supporting your body's immune system and lead to an improvement in inflammatory status. But a nutritional supplement should not be used as a substitute for a varied diet

Proper nutrition is essential in keeping your musculoskeletal (MSK) system operating to its full potential. If you are seeking chiropractic care to recover from an injury or just to maintain MSK health, nutrition becomes even more important.

Watch Your Caloric Intake

Although it has almost become cliché to talk about caloric intake, the foods you put in your body can go a long way in prolonging an MSK issue or putting extra strain on your muscles or joints. The more high caloric foods you eat, the more weight you're going to gain. The more weight you gain, the more pressure your muscle or joints come under. It's simple logic really, that most don't think about.

Tailored Diets

Your chiropractor has the education and expertise to tailor a diet or suggest foods that can directly address your injury or lifestyle.

For instance, those suffering from pain in a muscle or joint may be given an anti-inflammatory diet that avoids foods like white bread and french fries. These foods are recognized as a foreign invader by the body, leading to an increase in inflammation as well as a host of other problems.

Few Reciepes to keep in mind to help reduce pain

Kalamata Stuffed Chicken with Roasted Pepper Cream

(makes 6 servings)

Ingredients:

6 skinless boneless chicken breast halves

1/2 teaspoon freshly ground black pepper

2 oz. Sharp Cheddar, grated (1/2 cup)

1/2 whole wheat dry breadcrumbs

Cooking Spray

1 (7oz.) jar roasted red bell peppers, drained and patted dry

1/2 cup Plain Greek style Yogurt

1/4 teaspoon salt

Mixed salad greens

Preheat oven to 350 F

Place chicken between two sheets plastic wrap: pound with meat mallet or heavy pan to flatten. Uncover and sprinkle evenly with salt and peppers.

Sprinkle cheese and olives evenly onto center of each chicken breast; roll up, jellyroll-style and secure with wooden toothpicks. Dredge chicken rolls in breadcrumbs.

Place rolls seam-side down on baking sheet coated with cooking spray; lighty coat with cooking spray. Bake for 25-30 minutes or until chicken is cooked all the way to center

Meanwhile, pulse red peppers in food processor until pureed; add yogurt and salt, pulshing just untilsmooth. Refrigerate until ready to serve.

Remove chicken from oven and remove toothpicks. Let cool slightly. Slice; into 1-in. thick slices; arrange over salad green and serve with red bell peppers sauce.

Gluten Free Pancakes

(1 Dozen 5- Inch pancakes)

Ingredients

1 cup gluten Free cake flour

2 teaspoons baking powder

2 tablespoons sugar

1/2 teaspoon salt

1 egg

1/2 to 3/4 cup milk

2 tablespoon butter (melted & cooked

Sift cake flour, baking powder, sugar & salt

Beat egg & add butter

Add egg mixture to flour

Add milk until desired thickness

Stir only enough to moisten mixture.

Heat griddle & lightly grease it

Spoon batter onto griddle & coook until surface is dooted with holes. Flip & cook until light brown

Keep all pancakes warm in 200 F oven until serving

Homemade Granola

Ingredients:

5 cups of Rolled Oats

1 tbsp. cinnamon

1/4 tsp. SVA Super Spice #3

1 half tsp. stevia

1 third cup vegetable oil

1 cup raw sunflower seeds

1 cup raw pumpkin seeds

1 1/2 cups dried fruit

1/4 cup of honey

Directions:

Combine oats, cinnamon, stevia, and SVA spice in large bowl. Preheat oven to 350 degrees. Slowly pour oil into mixture and stir to coat evenly. Line two cookie sheets with aluminum foil and spread mixture evenly and pat down. Bake for 30 minutes flipping mixture half way through. When finished turn off oven. Microwave honey for 30 seconds on high until fluid. Gather seeds and dried fruit and when granola is cooked, combine all ingredients into large mixing bowl and slowly pour the honey into mix evenly coating. Transfer the mixture to cookie sheets and store in oven overnight

Blackberry Nectarine Crisp

(Serves 12)

Ingredients:

Vegetable oil cooking spray

3 cup fresh blackberries

3 large nectarines, pitted and sliced

1/4 fresh orange juice

2 tsp pur vanilla extract

1/2 cup whole wheat flour

1/2 cup old-fashioned rolled oats

1/3 cup packed light brown sugar

3 tbsp canola oil

2 tbsp honey

1 tsp ground cinnamon

pinch of freshly grated nutmeg

fresh mint sprigs, for serving

Directions:

Preheat oven to 350 degrees F

Coat a 9-inch baking dish or twelve 4-ounce ramekins with cooking spray

In a large bowl, combine the blackberries, nectarines, orange juice, and vanilla. Stir gently until well combined. Set aside.

In a separate bowl, sift the flour. Add the oats, brown sugar, canola oil, honey, cinnamon, and nutmeg. Use your hands to mix the ingredients until well blended.

Spoon the fruit mixture into the prepared baking dish, and scatter the crumb mixture evenly over the fruit.

Bake until the fruit bubbles, and the crumb topping is golden brown, 15 to 20 minutes for individual ramekins, or 30 minutes for a single large dish.

Place each ramekin on a small plate, or spoon the crisp onto 12 small plates.

Garnish each serving with 1 or 2 nectarine slices and a sprig of fresh mint. Serve hot.

Colorful Vegetable Pasta

(Serves 4)

Ingredients:

2 cups cooked spaghetti noodles (try Soba, Dreamfields, rice or wholegrain) drained

4 carrots

1 large zucchini

1 large summer squash

1 cup sprouted lentils or garbanzo beans, or 1 1/4 cup canned, drained, rinsed

1/4 cup chopped, sundried or cherry tomatoes

2 garlic cloves peeled and mashed

1/4 cup olive oil

zest of 1 lemon

juice of 2 lemons

1/4 cup chopped fresh basil or 1/2 tablespoon dried basil

1/2 tablespoon chopped fresh oregano or 1 teaspoon dried oregano

Directions:

Using a julienne or vegetable peeler, make long peels from the carrots, zucchini and summer squash.

If you prefer softer vegetables, add the julienne vegetables to the last 1 minute of cook time of pasta.

Add garlic, olive oil, zest and juice to a bowl. Stir, add pasta and julienne vegetables. Toss.

Add pasta to serving platter and top with lentils, tomatoes and herbs.

Cauliflower Couscous

(Serves 4)

Ingredients:

1 small head cauliflower, trim by cutting off stems with only florets remaining

1/8 cup olive oil

1/4 cup finely chopped purple cabbage

1/4 cup finely chopped carrots

1/4 cup finely chopped sundried or cherry tomatoes

1/4 cup finely chopped red onion

2 garlic cloves peeled and mashed

zest of 1/2 lime

juice of 1 lime

2 tablespoons of chopped cilantro leaves or try parsley, basil, marjoram or savory

1 tablespoon chia seeds

Directions:

Place raw cauliflower in a food processor, pulse until it resembles couscous.

Add to a bowl and stir in remaining ingrediants.

If a softer couscous is desired, place processed cauliflower in a fine mesh strainer, place over a pot filled with 2" of water, bring to a boil, cover and steam for 3 minutes or desired tenderness.

Veggie Fried Black Rice

(Serves 4)

Ingredients:

2 T water

1 tsp sesame oil

1 medium onion, diced

1 cup diced carrot

1 tsp minced garlic

1 tsp peeled and minced fresh ginger

1/2 cup frozen peas

1/2 cup frozen corn

1/2 cup diced red bell pepper

2 tsp wheat-free tamari

3 cups cooked Lotus Foods Forbidden Black Rice

1/2 cup sliced scallions, for garnish

1/2 cup roasted peanuts, for garnish

Directions:

Heat the water and oil in a large skillet over medium heat. Add the onion, carrot, garlic, and ginger and cook and stir for 5 minutes.

Add the peas, corn, bell pepper, and a few drops of tamari. Cook and stir for 5 minutes.

Spoon the rice on top of the cooked vegetables in the skillet and sprinkle the remaining tamari. Cover and cook over medium heat for 5 minutes, or until the rice is warm and the vegetables are tender. Stir before serving. Serve hot, garnished with the scallions and peanuts

Healthy Oatmeal

Ingredients:

1 cup oatmeal steel oats

2 cup hot water

1/8 cup chopped walnuts

1/3 cup dried cranberries

1/8 tsp cinnamon

Directions:

Bring water to a boil, add oats, reduce heat and cover 12-18 min, remove heat, let stand for a few minutes, 2-3 servings. Pour into bowls and add fruits, nuts, and sprinkle with cinnamon.

Lifestyle nutrition is also something your chiropractor can assist you with. If you or your child are into athletics a diet rich in complex carbohydrates is essential to provide the energy source to fuel your intense training and competition. Your chiropractor can assist you in developing a meal plan to meet your needs.

As your chiropractor I have the necessary training to provide you with nutritional advice in conjunction with your chiropractic treatment. Students on the road to becoming DCs (Doctors of Chiropractic) will receive classes in physiology, biochemistry and nutrition as part of the core curriculum. Together, with other courses that focus on a healthy lifestyle and whole-body wellness strategies, as your chiropractor I am an excellent resource to assist you in your ⬚uest for healthy choices and better all-around health.

Book an apointment with Dr Shaun Ang today at chiropractic concepts pte ltd (Singapore) for your chiropractic consultations and treatment.

Conclusion

Protective tension in a muscle develops for various reasons and must be examined accordingly. At GP, our assessments are used to identify protective tension and why it is present. This provides us with the information needed to design the most appropriate course of treatment and client education.

Disclaimer

The information contained within this eBook is strictly for educational purposes. If you wish to apply ideas contained in this eBook, you are taking full responsibility for your actions.

The author has made every effort to ensure the accuracy of the information within this book was correct at time of publication. The author does not assume and hereby disclaims any liability to any party for any loss, damage, or disruption caused by errors or omissions, whether such errors or omissions result from accident, negligence, or any other cause. (medical, Chiropractic)

Do not go yet; One last thing to do

If you enjoyed this book or found it useful I'd be very grateful if you'd post a short review on it. Your support really does make a difference and I read all the reviews personally so I can get your feedback and make this book even better.

Thanks again for your support!

www.ingramcontent.com/pod-product-compliance
Lightning Source LLC
Chambersburg PA
CBHW020613220526
45463CB00006B/2571